CHAIR YOGA WORKOUT FOR SENIORS OVER 60

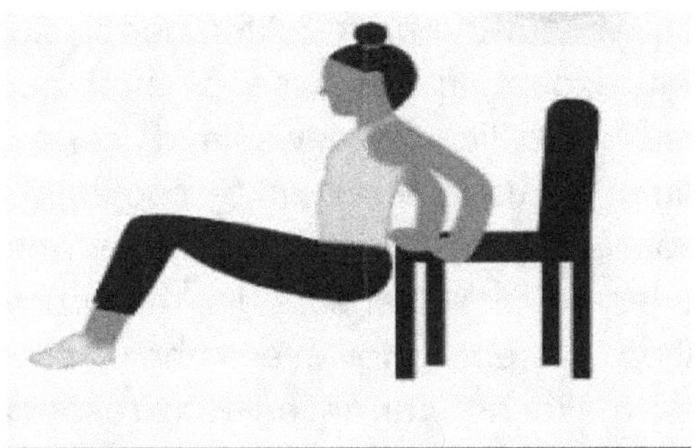

10-minutes illustrated Exercise to Improve your core Strength, Balance and Flexibility for a Healthier Independence Lifestyle

REITZ PRESCOTT

TABLE OF CONTENTS

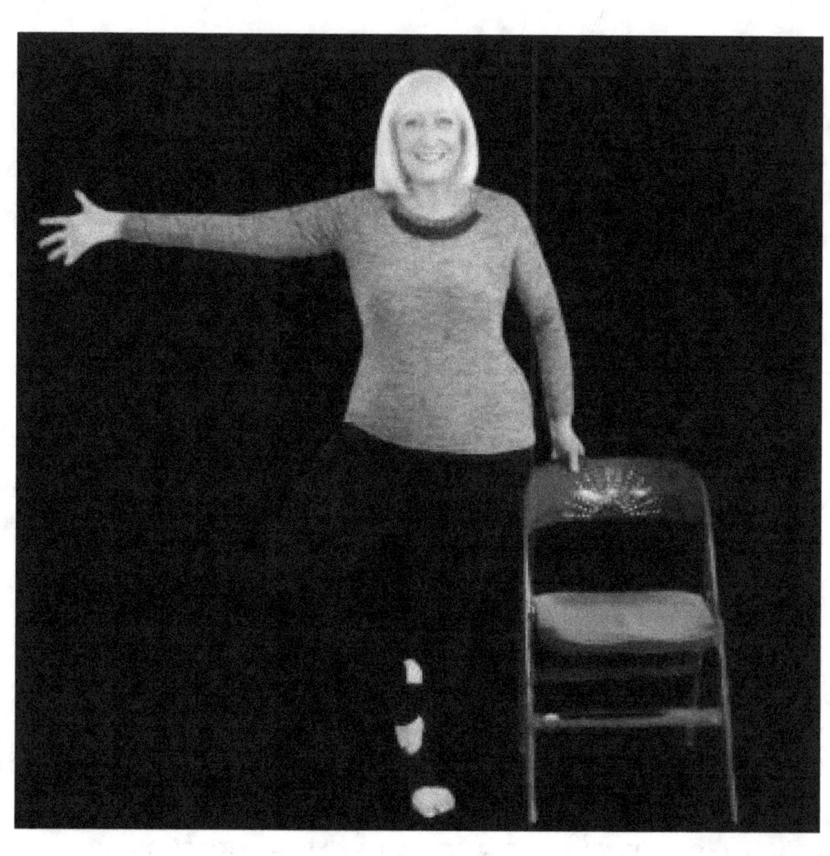

How to use this book

This complete book "Chair Yoga Workout for Seniors Over 60" offers accessible yoga practices to improve the physical and emotional health of senior citizens. The book provides clear and easy-to-follow instructions for incorporating yoga into a daily routine while seated in a chair, making it an ideal resource for seniors looking to improve flexibility, strength, and overall health.

The guide begins with an introduction to the benefits of chair yoga, emphasizing its gentle nature and suitability for individuals with limited mobility. It includes a variety of exercises targeting different muscle groups, accompanied by detailed illustrations and step-by-step instructions. The routines focus on promoting joint flexibility, balance, and relaxation, addressing common concerns associated with aging.

Readers can tailor the workouts to their fitness levels, gradually progressing as they become more comfortable with the exercises. This book also emphasizes the importance of mindful breathing and meditation, fostering mental clarity and stress relief. With its user-friendly approach, "Chair Yoga Workout for Seniors Over 60" empowers older individuals to incorporate a rejuvenating yoga practice into their lives, promoting a healthier and more active lifestyle.

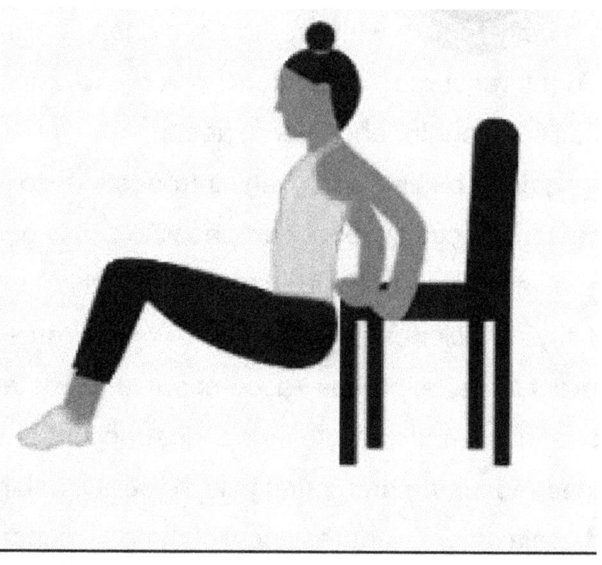

INTRODUCTION

Welcome to our Chair Yoga Workout for Seniors Over 60! As we age, it's essential to maintain flexibility, strength, and overall well-being. Chair yoga offers a gentle yet effective way to achieve these goals, catering specifically to the needs of seniors who may have limited mobility or balance concerns. Whether you're new to yoga or a seasoned practitioner, this program is designed to help you stay active, improve circulation, enhance flexibility, and promote relaxation—all from the comfort of a chair.

In this book session, we'll guide you through a series of gentle yoga poses and breathing exercises that can be easily adapted to your individual needs and abilities. You'll learn how to use the support of a chair to safely perform each movement, making this workout accessible to everyone, regardless of fitness level.

Before we begin, it's essential to listen to your body and honor its limitations. If you experience any discomfort or pain during the practice, please adjust the poses or skip them altogether. Remember, the goal is not perfection but rather progress and enjoyment.

Throughout the session, we'll focus on mindful breathing, which can help reduce stress, calm the mind, and improve concentration. So, let's take a moment to settle into our chairs, find a comfortable seated position, and bring our attention to our breath.

As we embark on this journey together, I encourage you to approach each pose with curiosity and kindness toward yourself. Let go of any expectations and simply enjoy the experience of moving and breathing in a way that nourishes both your body and spirit.

Now, let's begin our Chair Yoga Workout for Seniors Over 60 with a sense of openness, gratitude, and joy.

CHAPTER ONE. Understanding Chair Yoga

BENEFITS FOR SENIORS

1. Improved Flexibility: Chair yoga incorporates gentle stretches that help improve flexibility in the muscles and joints. This increased range of motion can enhance mobility and make daily activities easier and more comfortable.

2. Enhanced Strength: Despite being seated, chair yoga poses can still engage and strengthen various muscle groups, including the core, arms, legs, and back. Strengthening these muscles can help seniors maintain stability, prevent falls, and support overall physical function.

3. Better Balance and Stability: Chair yoga includes exercises that focus on balance and coordination, which are crucial for seniors to maintain independence and prevent falls. By practicing stability-enhancing poses regularly, seniors can improve their balance and reduce the risk of accidents.

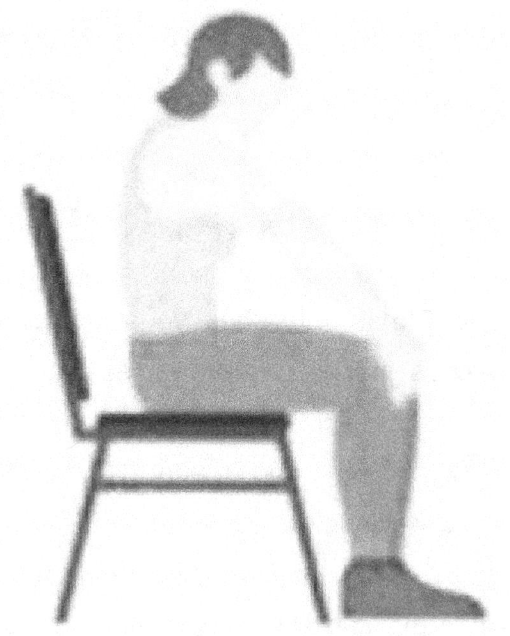

4. Increased Circulation: The gentle movements and deep breathing techniques in chair yoga can help improve blood circulation throughout the body. Enhanced circulation delivers oxygen and nutrients to cells more efficiently, promoting overall cardiovascular health and aiding in the healing process.

5. Stress Reduction and Relaxation: Chair yoga encourages mindfulness and relaxation through deep breathing and meditation techniques. By promoting relaxation and stress reduction, chair yoga can help seniors manage anxiety, improve sleep quality, and enhance overall mental well-being.

6. Pain Relief: Many seniors experience chronic pain, particularly in areas such as the back, hips, and joints. Chair yoga can help alleviate pain by gently stretching and strengthening the muscles surrounding these areas, promoting better alignment and reducing discomfort.

7. Improved Posture: Poor posture is common among seniors and can contribute to back pain, decreased mobility, and reduced quality of life. Chair yoga emphasizes proper alignment and encourages seniors to sit and stand with awareness, ultimately improving posture and spinal health.

8. Social Interaction: Participating in a chair yoga class provides seniors with an opportunity to socialize and connect with others in a supportive and inclusive environment. Building social connections can help combat feelings of isolation and loneliness, contributing to overall emotional well-being.

Chair yoga offers a multitude of benefits for seniors over 60, supporting their physical, mental, and emotional health and promoting a higher quality of life. Whether you're looking to increase flexibility, strengthen muscles, or simply unwind and relax, chair yoga provides a gentle yet effective way to stay active and healthy as you age.

TAILORING YOGA FOR SENIORS NEEDS

As we embark on this chair yoga journey designed specifically for seniors over 60, it's essential to recognize and address the unique needs of this demographic. Tailoring yoga for seniors involves thoughtful modifications and considerations to ensure a safe, enjoyable, and beneficial experience. Here's how we customize our chair yoga sessions to cater to the specific needs of our senior participants:

1.Adaptive Poses and Movements:

- Modify traditional yoga poses to accommodate any physical limitations or discomfort.
- Focus on poses that can be comfortably performed while seated or with the support of a chair.
- Offer variations and encourage participants to adapt poses to their comfort level.

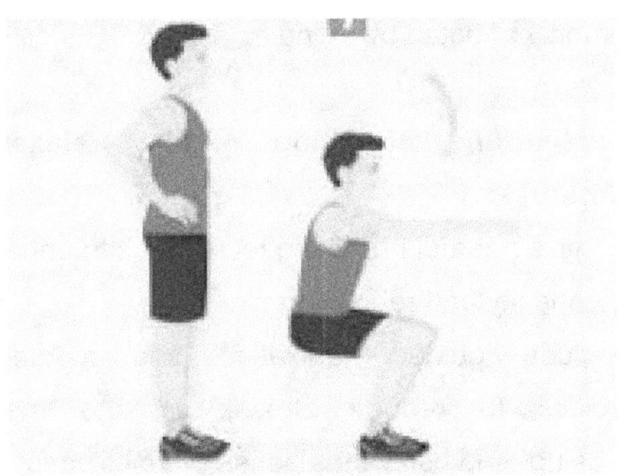

2. Chair as a Supportive Prop: Utilize the chair as a stable and supportive prop throughout the practice.

- Integrate the chair for balance in standing poses, as a tool for seated stretches, and as a helpful aid for movements requiring support.

3. Gentle Warm-ups and Joint Mobility:

- Begin each session with gentle warm-up exercises to prepare the body for movement.

- Incorporate joint mobility exercises to promote flexibility and ease stiffness, especially in areas commonly affected by aging.

4. Mindful Breathing and Relaxation Techniques:

- Prioritize mindful breathing techniques to enhance lung capacity and relaxation.

- Include guided relaxation and meditation exercises to reduce stress, promote mental well-being, and cultivate a sense of inner peace.

5. Slow and Controlled Movements:- Emphasize slow and controlled movements to prevent strain and reduce the risk of injury.

- Encourage participants to move at their own pace, fostering a mindful connection between body and breath.

6. Focus on Core Strength and Stability:

- Incorporate exercises that target core strength to support overall stability and balance.

- Strengthening the core muscles aids in maintaining an upright posture and preventing falls.

7. Joint-Friendly Practices:

- Integrate movements that are gentle on the joints, such as low-impact exercises that promote joint health.

 - Avoid abrupt or high-impact movements that may cause discomfort.

8. Encourage Social Interaction:

- Foster a sense of community by encouraging social interaction during sessions.

- Create an inclusive and supportive environment where participants can share experiences and build connections.

9. Individualized Attention:

- Provide individualized guidance, addressing the unique needs and concerns of each participant.
- Offer modifications or alternatives for participants with specific physical conditions.

10. Safety First:

- Prioritize safety by ensuring that participants use sturdy chairs placed on a non-slip surface.
- Remind participants to listen to their bodies and not push beyond their comfort levels.

CHAPTER TWO
Exercises for Strength and Flexibility

GENTLE WARM-UP AND STRENGTHEN MOVES

Warm-Up:

Neck and Shoulder Rolls

Begin your chair yoga practice with gentle neck and shoulder rolls to release tension and improve mobility. Place your feet firmly on the floor and settle into your chair. Inhale deeply as you gently roll your neck from side to side, feeling the release of tension in your neck and shoulders. Repeat this movement several times, focusing on the smoothness and fluidity of the motion.

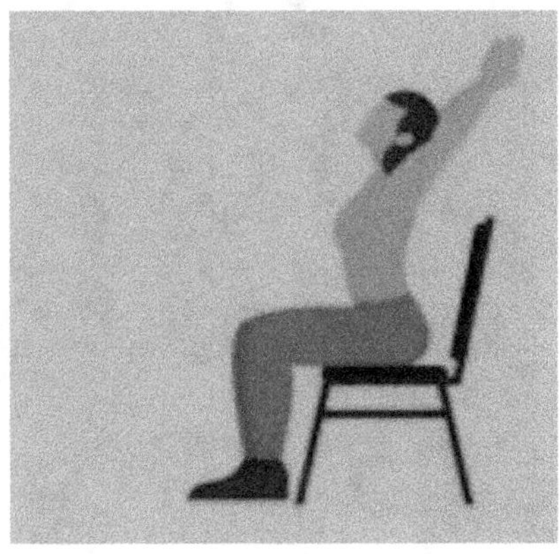

Arm and Wrist Stretches

Next, move on to arm and wrist stretches to enhance flexibility and strength in these areas. Extend your arms out to the sides, palms facing forward, and gently rotate your wrists in circular motions. Feel the stretch in your wrists, forearms, and shoulders. Continue with simple arm stretches, reaching one arm overhead and gently pulling the elbow with the opposite hand to deepen the stretch.

Leg Stretches for Stability

Shift your focus to leg stretches to enhance stability and mobility. Sitting firmly on the chair, extend one leg straight out in front of you, flexing the foot. Hold the position for a few breaths, feeling the stretch along the back of the leg. Switch to the other leg and repeat. This exercise helps improve flexibility in the hamstrings and promotes better balance.

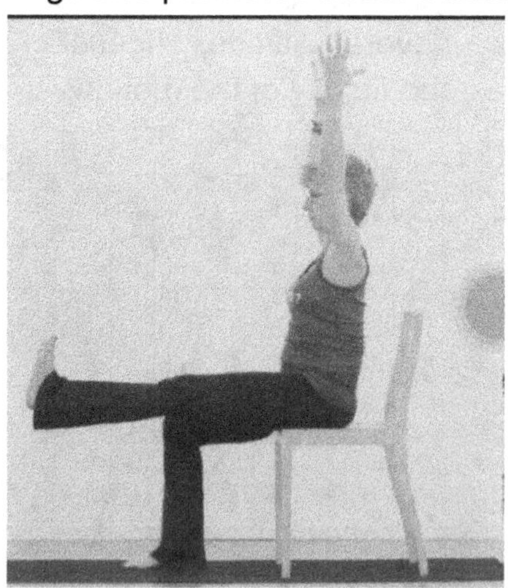

Core Engaging Mountain Pose

Transition into a seated version of Mountain Pose to engage your core and improve posture. Sit tall on your chair with feet flat on the floor. Inhale as you reach your arms overhead, palms facing each other. Engage your core by drawing your navel towards your spine. Feel the lengthening of your spine and the activation of your abdominal muscles. Hold the pose for a few breaths, focusing on your alignment and breathing.

Seated Forward Bend

Continue with a gentle Seated Forward Bend to stretch your spine and hamstrings while strengthening your core. Sit upright on the edge of your chair with feet hip-width apart. Inhale to lengthen your spine, then exhale as you hinge at the hips to fold forward, reaching towards your feet or shins. Avoid curving your spine by maintaining a straight back.   Feel the gentle stretch along the back of your legs and hold for a few breaths before slowly returning to an upright position.

These gentle warm-up exercises and strengthening poses are designed to prepare the body for the chair yoga practice, promoting flexibility, mobility, and stability for seniors over 60. Feel free to adapt these exercises to suit individual needs and comfort levels, emphasizing smooth, controlled movements and mindful breathing throughout the practice.

SEATED YOGA POSES FOR FLEXIBILITY AND STRENGTH

Seated Side Stretch

Commence with a Seated Side Stretch to enhance flexibility in the torso and promote spinal mobility.Place your feet flat on the floor and sit tall in the chair. Reach your right arm overhead, inhale, and as you exhale, gently lean to the left, feeling the stretch along the right side of your body. Hold the stretch for a few breaths, then return to center and repeat on the other side. Embrace the gentle lengthening of your side body with each breath.

Seated Leg Extension Pose

Transition into the Seated Leg Extension Pose to strengthen the quadriceps and promote flexibility in the hamstrings. Position yourself at the chair's edge, keeping your back straight. Extend one leg in front of you, flexing the foot. Hold the pose for a few breaths, feeling the engagement in your extended leg and the stretch in your hamstring.

Switch legs and repeat on the other side. Focus on maintaining an upright posture throughout the pose.

Seated Cow Face Pose Arms

Engage in the Seated Cow Face Pose for a delightful shoulder and arm stretch. Sit comfortably on the chair and extend your right arm overhead, bending it to reach behind your neck. Bring your left arm behind your back and try to clasp fingers or hold a towel between the hands. Feel the stretch in your shoulders and arms as you gently lift your chest. Hold for a few breaths, then switch arms to balance the stretch on both sides.

Seated Pigeon Pose Variation

Explore a Seated Pigeon Pose Variation to open up the hips and release tension in the lower back. Sit on the chair with your ankle resting on your opposite knee. Flex the foot of the ankle that is lifted to protect the knee. Sit tall, gently press on the lifted knee to deepen the stretch, feeling a soothing release in the hips and lower back. Hold the pose for a few breaths, then switch sides to balance the stretch.

Seated Boat Pose Variation

Engage in a Seated Boat Pose Variation to strengthen the core muscles and improve balance. Sit tall on the chair, lean back slightly, and lift your legs slightly off the floor, maintaining a straight back. For stability, cling to the chair's sides. Engage your core by drawing the navel towards the spine. Hold the pose for a few breaths, feeling the gentle activation of your abdominal muscles and the improvement in core strength.

These seated yoga poses are crafted to promote flexibility, strength, and balance for seniors over 60 within the framework of chair yoga. Embrace the fluidity of movement and the nurturing stretches to enhance your physical well-being and overall vitality. Modify poses as needed to suit your comfort level and enjoy the benefits of a regular chair yoga practice.

CHAPTER THREE
Mindful Breathing and Relaxation

DEEP BREATHING PRACTICE

Diaphragmatic Breathing (Deep Belly Breathing)
Commence your chair yoga practice with Diaphragmatic Breathing, also known as deep belly breathing, to promote relaxation and enhance oxygen flow. Sit comfortably on the chair with a straight back and place one hand on your chest and the other on your abdomen. Take a deep breath through your nose and feel your belly bubble up. As you slowly release the breath via your mouth, feel your belly constrict. Focus on the sensation of your breath moving in and out of your body, fostering a sense of calm and centeredness.

Box Breathing (Square Breathing)
Engage in Box Breathing, a methodical breathing technique that encourages relaxation and focus. Sit comfortably on the chair and begin by inhaling deeply for a count of four. Four counts are needed

to hold your breath at the peak of the inhale. Slowly exhale for a count of four, and then hold your breath at the bottom of the exhale for a count of four. Repeat this cycle several times, allowing each breath to flow smoothly and rhythmically. Box Breathing helps regulate the nervous system and promotes a sense of balance and tranquility.

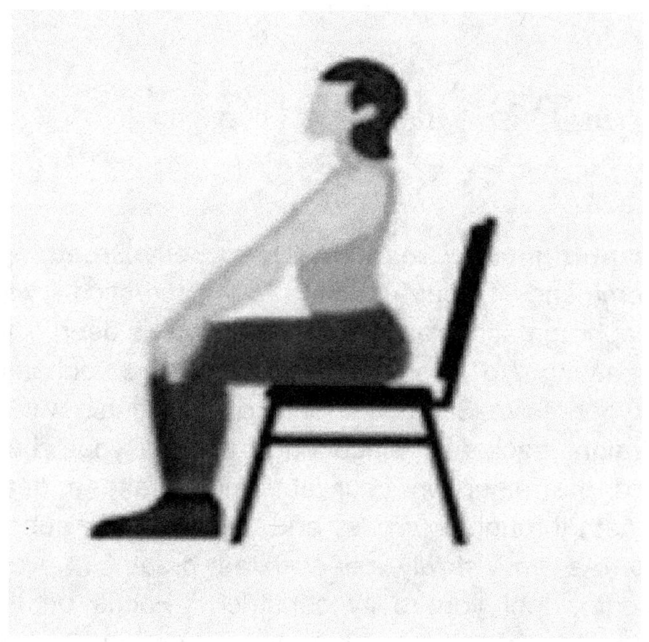

Alternate Nostril Breathing (Nadi Shodhana)
Explore Alternate Nostril Breathing, also known as Nadi Shodhana, to promote balance and clarity in the mind. Sit comfortably on the chair and place your left hand on your left knee. Raise your right hand and place your middle and index fingers in the

space between your eyebrows. Breathe deeply through your left nostril while closing your right nostril with your thumb. Close the left nostril with your ring finger, release the right nostril, and exhale through the right nostril. Inhale through the right nostril, close it, release the left nostril, and exhale through the left. Continue this cycle, allowing your breath to flow smoothly and evenly. Alternate Nostril Breathing helps harmonize the flow of energy in the body and fosters a sense of mental clarity and focus.

Three-Part Breath (Dirga Pranayama)
Engage in Three-Part Breath, also known as Dirga Pranayama, to deepen your breath capacity and cultivate relaxation. Sit comfortably on the chair, placing one hand on your abdomen and the other on your chest. Inhale deeply through your nose, first filling your abdomen, then your ribcage, and finally allowing your chest to expand. Exhale slowly and consciously, releasing the breath from your chest, ribcage, and abdomen. Focus on the sensation of your breath flowing through each part of your torso, nurturing a sense of groundedness and presence.

Cooling Breath (Sitali Pranayama)
Embrace Cooling Breath, also known as Sitali Pranayama, to promote a sense of calm and coolness in the body. Sit comfortably on the chair and curl your tongue into a "U" shape or purse your lips. Inhale slowly and deeply through your curled

tongue or pursed lips, feeling the coolness of the breath as it enters your body. Exhale gently through your nose. If you are unable to curl your tongue, simply purse your lips and inhale slowly through the small opening. Continue this cooling breath practice for several rounds, allowing it to soothe and refresh your mind and body.

These deep breathing practices are tailored to enhance relaxation, focus, and overall well-being for seniors over 60 within the setting of chair yoga. Embrace the transformative power of deep breathing, allowing each breath to guide you towards a state of calm and mental clarity. Feel free to integrate these practices into your chair yoga routine, nurturing a sense of balance and inner peace with each mindful breath.

GUIDED RELAXATION TECHNIQUES

Body Scan Relaxation

Begin your guided relaxation with a Body Scan practice to promote a sense of deep relaxation and body awareness. Sit comfortably on the chair, close your eyes, and bring your attention to your toes. Slowly move your focus up through each part of your body, from your feet to your head, noticing any sensations or areas of tension. With each breath, visualize releasing any tension or discomfort, allowing a wave of relaxation to wash over each body part. Embrace a sense of tranquility and presence as you journey through your body with mindful awareness.

Progressive Muscle Relaxation

Engage in Progressive Muscle Relaxation to release tension and enhance relaxation throughout your body. Sit comfortably on the chair and begin by gently tensing the muscles in your toes for a few seconds, then release the tension, feeling the relaxation flood in. Progressively move through each muscle group, from your feet to your forehead, alternating between tensing and releasing, allowing each area to soften and unwind. Embrace the contrast between tension and relaxation, fostering a deep sense of ease and tranquility within your body.

Guided Imagery

Explore Guided Imagery as a way to promote relaxation and mental calmness. Sit comfortably on the chair, close your eyes, and envision a peaceful and serene place in your mind's eye. It could be a tranquil beach, a lush forest, or a cozy spot by a crackling fireplace. Engage your senses as you visualize the sights, sounds, and smells of this imaginary sanctuary. Allow yourself to fully immerse in the imagery, feeling a deep sense of peace and rejuvenation wash over you. Embrace the restorative power of your mind to create a space of relaxation and tranquility.

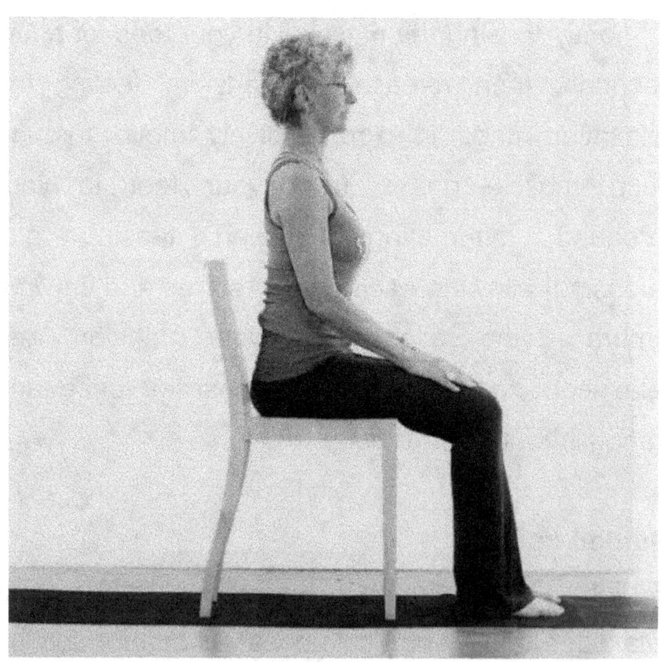

Breath Awareness Meditation

Engage in Breath Awareness Meditation to cultivate mindfulness and inner calm. Sit comfortably on the chair, close your eyes, and bring your focus to your breath. As your breath comes in and goes out of your body, pay attention to its organic rhythm. With each inhale and exhale, let go of any distracting thoughts or worries, allowing yourself to be fully present in the moment. Embrace the gentle rise and fall of your breath, feeling a sense of grounding and relaxation with each mindful breath. Allow the simplicity of your breath to guide you towards a state of inner peace and serenity.

Body Relaxation Visualization

Conclude your guided relaxation with a Body Relaxation Visualization to promote a sense of overall well-being and calm. Sit comfortably on the chair and envision a warm, golden light wrapping around your body, starting from your head and gradually moving down to your toes. Visualize this healing light gently enveloping each body part, soothing away any remaining tension or discomfort. Feel the warmth and comfort of this light as it nurtures your entire being, leaving you with a profound sense of relaxation and inner harmony.

These guided relaxation techniques are designed to foster a sense of deep relaxation, tranquility, and rejuvenation for seniors over 60 during their chair yoga practice. Embrace the restorative power of these practices, allowing them to nurture your body, mind, and spirit with each calming breath and gentle visualization. Incorporate these guided relaxation techniques into your chair yoga routine to cultivate a sense of peace and well-being throughout your practice.

CHAPTER FOUR
Integration into Daily Life

Assessing Your Needs

Begin by assessing your individual needs and goals for your chair yoga practice. Consider any areas of stiffness, weakness, or discomfort in your body that you would like to address. Evaluate your mobility, balance, and flexibility levels to tailor your routine accordingly.

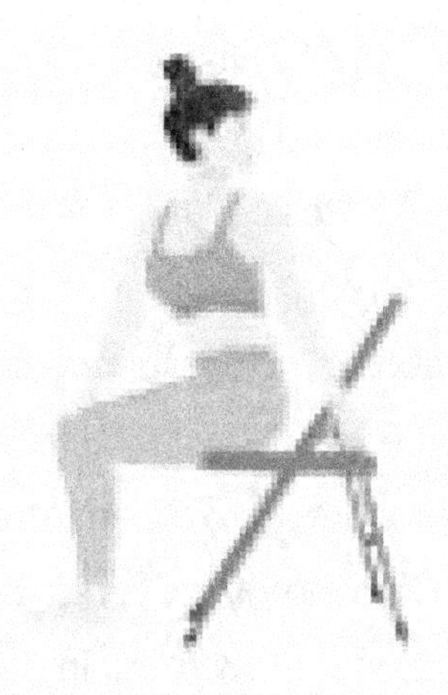

Gentle Warm-Up

Start your personalized chair yoga routine with a gentle warm-up to prepare your body for movement. Incorporate neck rolls, shoulder shrugs, and wrist circles to loosen up the joints and release tension. Focus on smooth, controlled movements to gradually increase blood flow and flexibility.

Seated Poses for Flexibility

Include a variety of seated poses that focus on enhancing flexibility in different areas of your body. Choose poses like Seated Forward Bend, Seated Twist, and Seated Side Stretch to stretch and lengthen your muscles, improve range of motion, and promote joint health.

Strengthening Poses

Incorporate strengthening poses to build muscle tone and stability. Include poses like Seated Warrior II, Seated Leg Lifts, and Seated Boat Pose to engage your core, legs, and arms. Strengthening exercises help improve overall body strength and support functional movement in daily activities.

Balancing Poses

Integrate balancing poses to challenge your stability and improve coordination. Poses like Seated Tree Pose, Seated Extended Hand-To-Big-Toe Pose, and Seated Knee to Chest pose are great for enhancing balance and proprioception. Focus on your breath and inner focus to maintain stability in these poses.

Breathing Practices

Include deep breathing exercises throughout your routine to promote relaxation and mindfulness. Incorporate techniques like Diaphragmatic Breathing, Box Breathing, and Alternate Nostril Breathing to enhance lung capacity, reduce stress, and improve mental clarity. Breathing practices can be interspersed between poses for a calming effect.

Cool Down and Relaxation

Conclude your personalized chair yoga routine with a calming cool-down and guided relaxation. Transition into gentle stretches like Seated Cat-Cow Stretch and Seated Child's Pose to release tension in the body.

Finish with a few moments of guided relaxation or meditation to unwind and restore a sense of peace and tranquility.

Modifications and Self-Care

Remember to listen to your body throughout your practice and modify poses as needed to suit your comfort level. Stay hydrated, take breaks when necessary, and honor your body's limitations. Embrace self-care practices like gentle self-massage, restorative poses, and mindful reflection to nourish your body and mind.

Consistency and Progression

Commit to a regular chair yoga practice to experience the full benefits of your personalized routine. Monitor your progress, celebrate small achievements, and gradually increase the intensity and duration of your practice as you build strength, flexibility, and confidence. Embrace the journey with patience and self-kindness as you discover the transformative power of chair yoga for seniors over 60.

By crafting a personalized chair yoga routine that suits your unique needs and preferences, you can tailor your practice to support your physical, mental, and emotional well-being. Enjoy the journey of self-discovery and empowerment as you embark on your chair yoga practice tailored specifically for seniors over 60.

FOSTERING INDEPENDENCE AND CONFERENCE

Empowering Mind-Body Connection

Chair yoga serves as a powerful tool for fostering independence and confidence in seniors over 60 by enhancing the mind-body connection. Through gentle movements, breath awareness, and mindfulness practices, individuals can cultivate a deeper understanding and appreciation of their bodies. This heightened awareness empowers seniors to take control of their physical well-being and make conscious choices that support their overall health.

Building Physical Strength and Stability

Engaging in chair yoga enables seniors to build physical strength and stability, which are essential components of independence. By incorporating strengthening poses and balance exercises into their practice, seniors can enhance muscle tone, improve posture, and boost confidence in their physical abilities. As strength and stability increase, daily tasks and activities become more manageable, leading to a greater sense of self-assurance and autonomy.

Enhancing Flexibility and Mobility

Chair yoga facilitates the improvement of flexibility and mobility, key factors in maintaining independence as we age. Through gentle stretching and joint mobilization exercises, seniors can increase range of motion, reduce stiffness, and enhance overall mobility. As flexibility improves, individuals feel more capable and empowered to move freely and engage in daily activities with confidence and ease.

Promoting Emotional Well-Being

Emotional well-being plays a vital role in fostering independence and confidence in seniors. Chair yoga provides a safe space for individuals to cultivate a sense of inner peace, relaxation, and emotional resilience. Through guided relaxation techniques, breath awareness, and meditation practices, seniors can manage stress, reduce anxiety, and nurture a positive mindset. This emotional stability translates into increased self-assurance and a greater sense of autonomy.

Encouraging Self-Care and Self-Compassion

Chair yoga promotes self-care and self-compassion, encouraging seniors to prioritize their well-being and listen to their bodies. By honoring their physical limitations, practicing mindfulness, and acknowledging their accomplishments, individuals can develop a deeper sense of self-acceptance and confidence. This self-awareness and self-compassion form the foundation for building independence and resilience in all aspects of life.

Cultivating a Sense of Achievement

Engagement in chair yoga enables seniors to set and achieve personal goals, leading to a sense of accomplishment and pride. By progressing in their practice, mastering new poses, and observing improvements in strength and flexibility, individuals develop a heightened sense of self-efficacy and belief in their abilities. This sense of achievement fosters independence and confidence, empowering seniors to navigate life's challenges with courage and determination.

Embracing Lifelong Learning and Growth

Chair yoga encourages seniors to embrace lifelong learning and personal growth by exploring new movement patterns, breathing techniques, and relaxation practices. By remaining curious, open-minded, and dedicated to their practice, individuals can continue to evolve physically, mentally, and emotionally. This commitment to growth instills a sense of resilience, independence, and confidence that transcends age and empowers seniors to live life to the fullest.

Embracing Independence with Every Breath

As seniors over 60 engage in chair yoga practice, they embark on a journey of self-discovery, self-empowerment, and self-expression. Through the nurturing environment of chair yoga, individuals can foster independence, confidence, and a profound sense of self-assurance. With each breath, each movement, and each moment of mindfulness, seniors harness the transformative power of chair yoga to cultivate a life filled with vitality, strength, and unwavering independence.

Empowering seniors over 60 through chair yoga practice not only fosters physical well-being but also nurtures a deep sense of independence, confidence, and self-empowerment. By embracing the holistic benefits of chair yoga, individuals can embark on a journey of self-discovery, growth, and resilience that fuels a life of purpose, vitality, and fulfillment.

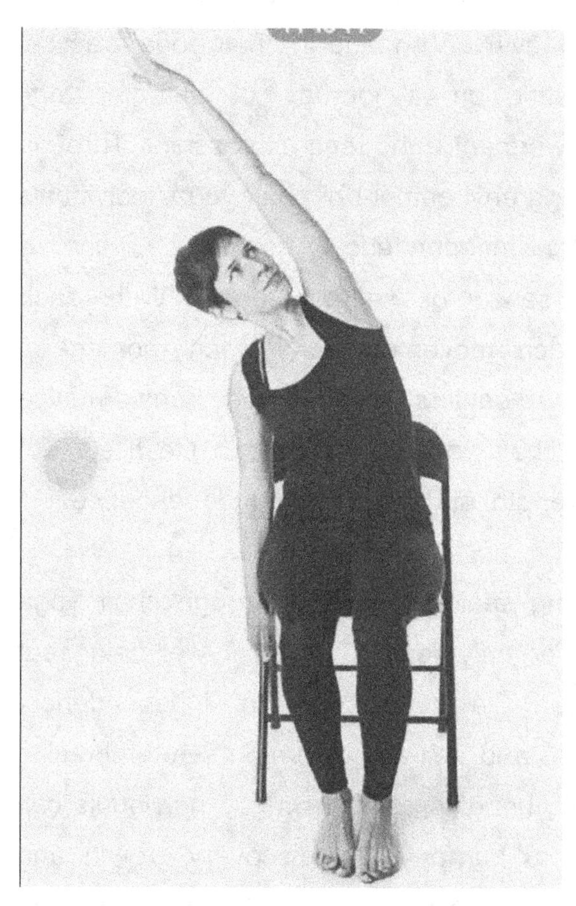

CHAPTER FIVE
Conclusion

Embracing Wellness and Vitality with Chair Yoga

As we bring our chair yoga workout for seniors over 60 to a close, it is essential to reflect on the transformative journey we have shared. Through the gentle movements, mindful breathwork, and nurturing practices of chair yoga, we have delved deep into the wellspring of well-being, vitality, and self-discovery. Chair yoga has served as a beacon of light, guiding us toward enhanced physical strength, flexibility, and balance. By embracing the practice with dedication and self-compassion, we have nurtured a deeper connection with our bodies, fostering resilience, independence, and confidence with each pose and breath.

Through guided relaxation techniques and mindfulness practices, we have crafted a sanctuary of peace and tranquility within ourselves. By tending to our emotional well-being and promoting self-care, we have cultivated a sense of inner calm and emotional resilience that transcends the boundaries of age.

Chair yoga has been a catalyst for personal growth, learning, and self-acceptance. By setting and achieving personal goals, embracing challenges with courage, and celebrating our achievements, we have fostered a sense of empowerment and self-assurance that resonates throughout our practice and daily lives.

As we conclude our chair yoga practice today, let us remember that well-being is a lifelong journey—a continuous exploration of self-discovery, growth, and resilience. By remaining committed to our practice, embracing the wisdom of our bodies, and fostering a sense of curiosity and openness, we pave the way for a future filled with vitality, strength, and unwavering independence.

In every breath, every movement, and every moment of mindful awareness, we embrace the transformative power of chair yoga. As we carry the lessons learned on our mats into our daily lives, let us embody the spirit of well-being, confidence, and vitality that chair yoga has instilled within us.

Gratitude and Connection

I **REITZ PRESCOTT** extend my heartfelt gratitude to each and every one of you for embarking on this chair yoga journey together. The laughter shared, the challenges embraced, and the moments of stillness and reflection have woven a tapestry of connection and shared growth that transcends physical boundaries.

With deep gratitude and a sense of shared purpose, I bid you farewell with a reverent . The light and divine essence within me honors the light and divine essence within each of you. May you continue to walk your path with courage, grace, and a heart filled with the boundless possibilities that chair yoga has revealed within you.

As we conclude our chair yoga practice today, may the lessons learned and the insights gained continue to shape your journey towards enhanced well-being, vitality, and unwavering self-assurance. Embrace the transformative power of chair yoga as a guiding light on your path to a life filled with joy, strength, and boundless possibility.

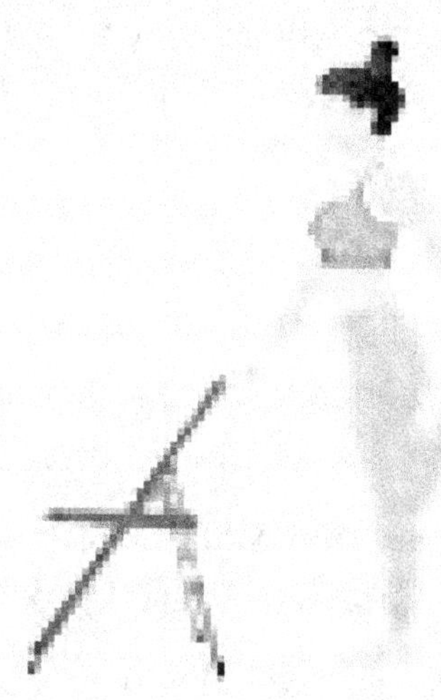

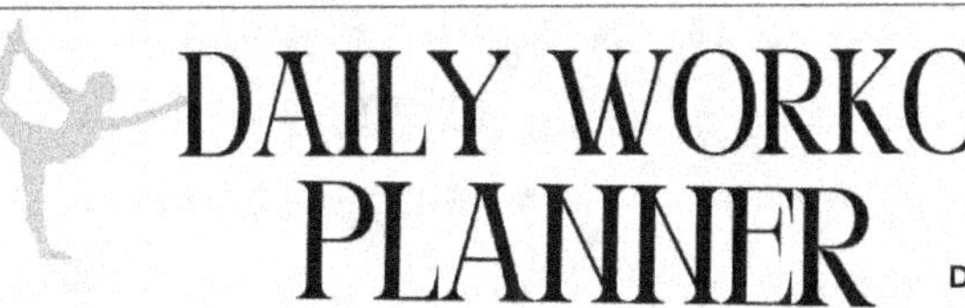
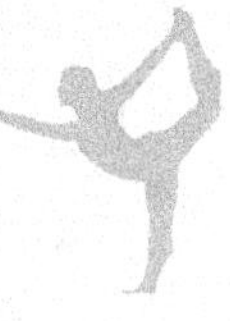

DAILY WORKOUT PLANNER

DATE

TODAY'S GOALS

WATER INTAKE

○ ○ ○
○ ○ ○

WORKOUT	**TIME**

MEAL PLAN

BREAKFAST

LUNCH

DINNER

"YOUR FITNESS PLANNER IS YOUR ROADMAP TO SUCCESS, GUIDING EACH STEP TOWARDS A HEALTHIER, STRONGER YOU."

NOTE

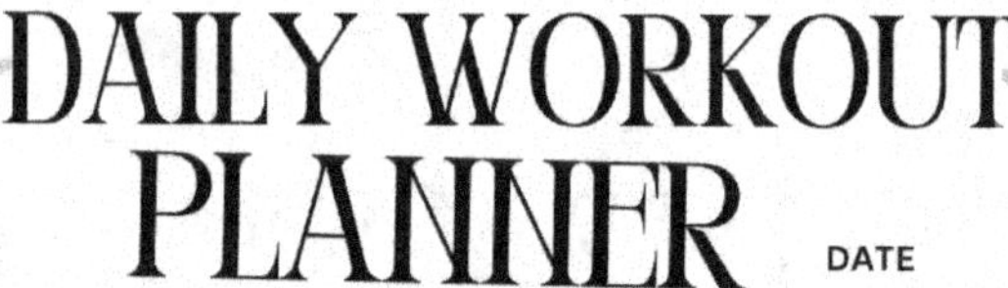

DAILY WORKOUT PLANNER

DATE

TODAY'S GOALS

WATER INTAKE

WORKOUT **TIME**

MEAL PLAN

BREAKFAST

LUNCH

DINNER

"YOUR FITNESS PLANNER IS YOUR ROADMAP TO SUCCESS, GUIDING EACH STEP TOWARDS A HEALTHIER, STRONGER YOU."

NOTE

DAILY WORKOUT PLANNER

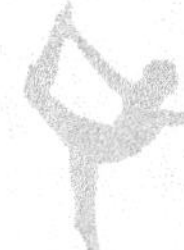

DATE

TODAY'S GOALS

WATER INTAKE

WORKOUT	TIME

MEAL PLAN

BREAKFAST

LUNCH

DINNER

"YOUR FITNESS PLANNER IS YOUR ROADMAP TO SUCCESS, GUIDING EACH STEP TOWARDS A HEALTHIER, STRONGER YOU."

NOTE

DAILY WORKOUT PLANNER

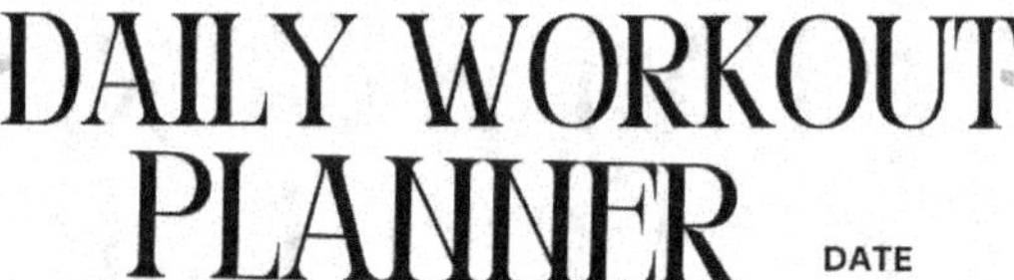

DATE

TODAY'S GOALS

WATER INTAKE

WORKOUT	TIME

MEAL PLAN

BREAKFAST

LUNCH

DINNER

NOTE

DAILY WORKOUT PLANNER

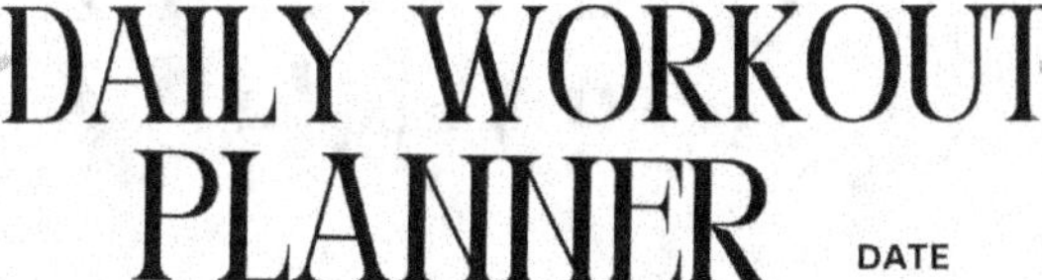

DATE

TODAY'S GOALS

WATER INTAKE

WORKOUT	TIME

MEAL PLAN

BREAKFAST

LUNCH

DINNER

"YOUR FITNESS PLANNER IS YOUR ROADMAP TO SUCCESS, GUIDING EACH STEP TOWARDS A HEALTHIER, STRONGER YOU."

NOTE

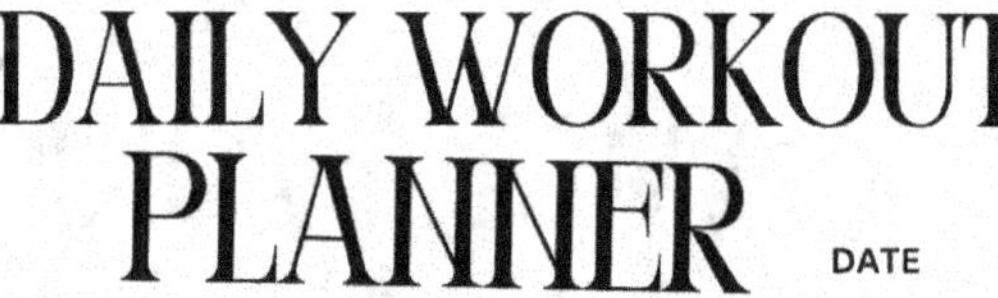

DAILY WORKOUT PLANNER

DATE

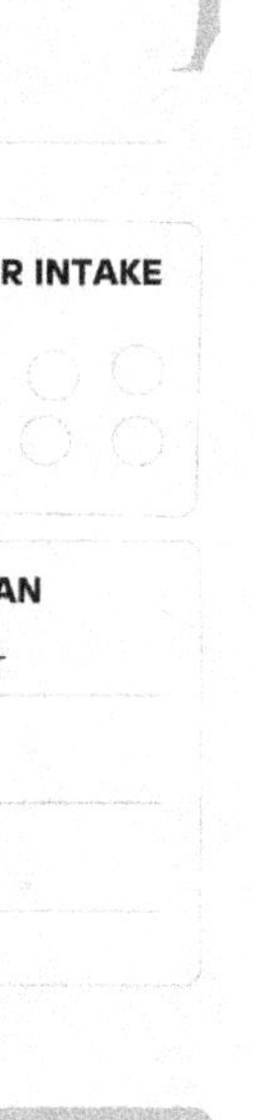

TODAY'S GOALS

WATER INTAKE

WORKOUT	TIME

MEAL PLAN

BREAKFAST

LUNCH

DINNER

NOTE

DAILY WORKOUT PLANNER

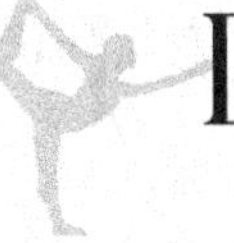

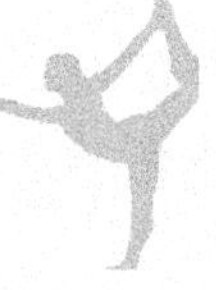

DATE

TODAY'S GOALS

WATER INTAKE

WORKOUT

TIME

MEAL PLAN

BREAKFAST

LUNCH

DINNER

"YOUR FITNESS PLANNER IS YOUR ROADMAP TO SUCCESS, GUIDING EACH STEP TOWARDS A HEALTHIER, STRONGER YOU."

NOTE

DAILY WORKOUT PLANNER

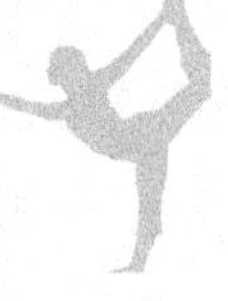

DATE

TODAY'S GOALS

WATER INTAKE

WORKOUT | **TIME**

MEAL PLAN

BREAKFAST

LUNCH

DINNER

"YOUR FITNESS PLANNER IS YOUR ROADMAP TO SUCCESS, GUIDING EACH STEP TOWARDS A HEALTHIER, STRONGER YOU."

NOTE

DAILY WORKOUT PLANNER

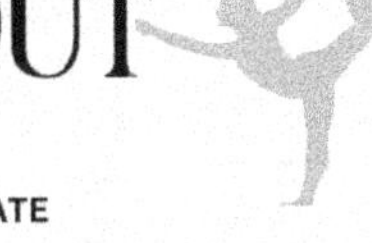

DATE

TODAY'S GOALS

WATER INTAKE

WORKOUT	TIME

MEAL PLAN

BREAKFAST

LUNCH

DINNER

"YOUR FITNESS PLANNER IS YOUR ROADMAP TO SUCCESS, GUIDING EACH STEP TOWARDS A HEALTHIER, STRONGER YOU."

NOTE

DAILY WORKOUT PLANNER

DATE

TODAY'S GOALS

WATER INTAKE

WORKOUT

TIME

MEAL PLAN

BREAKFAST

LUNCH

DINNER

"YOUR FITNESS PLANNER IS YOUR ROADMAP TO SUCCESS, GUIDING EACH STEP TOWARDS A HEALTHIER, STRONGER YOU."

NOTE